Eduardo Janir de Souza
Mariane Almeida

# Professional training for nurses through realistic simulation

Eduardo Janir de Souza
Mariane Almeida

# Professional training for nurses through realistic simulation

## Knowledge beyond books

ScienciaScripts

**Imprint**



Cover image: www.ingimage.com

This book is a translation from the original published under ISBN 978-613-9-69167-8.

Publisher:
Sciencia Scripts
is a trademark of
Dodo Books Indian Ocean Ltd. and OmniScriptum S.R.L publishing group

120 High Road, East Finchley, London, N2 9ED, United Kingdom
Str. Armeneasca 28/1, office 1, Chisinau MD-2012, Republic of Moldova, Europe
Printed at: see last page
**ISBN: 978-620-8-12599-8**

"Success is born of desire, determination and persistence in reaching a goal. Even if you don't reach the target, those who seek it out and overcome obstacles will at the very least do admirable things."

SUMMARY

The main objective of this work was to carry out a pedagogical practice that integrated the curricular components in an interdisciplinary way in order to stimulate meaningful and contextualised learning for students, through Active Methodologies in the Nursing course at the Universidade do Oeste de Santa Catarina - UNOESC - Campus de Joaçaba-SC, reflecting the precepts of the National Curriculum Guidelines for higher education courses, as well as those of the Unified Health System (SUS). It should be noted that the aim is to meet the prerogatives of the Nursing Course's Pedagogical Project, through multi/interdisciplinary practice, promoting multiple dialogues between the Structuring Teaching Group, the course collegiate body and students, in order to provide innovative teaching practices in the health area, as well as stimulating research, logical reasoning and meaningful learning on the part of the students. This activity involved around 70 per cent of the curricular components of the Nursing course, involving all stages of the course, totalling 174 students. The activity was devised at a meeting with the NDE and the Nursing course collegiate body at the Unoesc Joaçaba Campus, involving the teaching plan at the start of the semester for the curricular components and culminated in many activities, such as the presentation of a Realistic Simulation - Simulated Jury, PBL (Problem-Based Learning), round table discussion and others. The theme used was chosen by the course board - Mental Health - which analysed a fact involving a case with national repercussions concerning the situation of nursing. For three months, each of the curricular components involved tried to deal with and analyse the case across the board, reading articles, seminars, discussions, among others, as well as teaching methodologies in which the students actively participated in the process. The culmination of the activity was the presentation of the case by the seventh phase of the Nursing course. The result of the activities reported consolidates the multi/interdisciplinary projects for each academic semester, as well as improving pedagogical practice in nursing teaching and enabling meaningful learning for the students.

Keywords: Active Methodologies. Nursing Education. Mental Health. Autism.

**CONTENTS**

# CHAPTER 1

# INTRODUCTION

Until recently, the university was considered one of the only sources for disseminating knowledge, and people turned to it to acquire, update and specialise information.

Nowadays, the search for "knowledge" is not restricted to educational institutions alone, since we are subject to being surprised every day by new information available to students, which we don't always have the opportunity to see on the countless websites on the Internet, and the role of the teacher as a mere information relay is numbered.

This will reveal a pedagogical approach that is more committed to learning, as well as the use of active methodologies in the process of acquiring knowledge. In other words, pedagogical practices that lead academics to reflect on their practice.

To this end, realistic simulation contributes to the acquisition of a more confident attitude in future professionals, who will make strategically planned decisions for the benefit of all. According to (FREIRE, 2009), in addition to these aspects, this approach makes great contributions to the teaching and learning process, since it generates satisfaction for the student, who will test their knowledge beforehand, and for the teacher, who will be able to check the progress and effectiveness of their lessons.

Thinking about teaching practices in the Life Sciences area, more precisely in the nursing course, in times of such profound transformations, requires the audacity not to fit demands into old learning models and the lucidity to find their potential in concrete situations. From this perspective, we take on the challenge of outlining teaching practices from innovative perspectives, breaking with a culture of transmitting information and investing in problematising students' reality, configuring processes in which learning is understood as a social, historical practice conditioned by trajectories, knowledge and experiences (FREIRE, 2009).

The aim of this study is therefore to implement a pedagogical practice that integrates curricular components in an interdisciplinary way in order to stimulate meaningful and contextualised learning for students, using active methodologies in the Nursing course at the University of the West of Santa Catarina, Joaçaba Campus.

## 1.1 OBJECTIVES

### 1.1.1 General Objective

Carrying out a pedagogical practice that integrates curricular components in an interdisciplinary way in order to stimulate meaningful and contextualised student learning through active methodologies in the Nursing course at the Universidade do Oeste de Santa Catarina, Campus de Joaçaba- SC.

### 1.1.2 Specific objectives

- Estimular o ensino baseado em evidência through active methodologies in the Nursing course.
- Desenvolver Realistic simulation as an innovative pedagogical practice in the Nursing course.
- Promover a reflexão de práticas que estimulem o ensino e a learning through active methodologies.
- Promover situations of experience between teaching, research and the applicability of innovative pedagogical practices in the Nursing course.
- Qualificar as bases teóricas e metodológicas do ensino de graduação em Nursing with a focus on decision-making by students in practical situations in various health contexts.

### 1.1.3 Clarifying note

It should be emphasised that this work was prepared and written by six people, so many texts were shared, mainly in the theoretical background, as well as in the results. The difference in each work is related to the focus given by each participant in this project, since the starting point was the same, but the activities developed were different, in this case my final considerations will focus on the activities developed in the Mental Health discipline.

# CHAPTER 2

# RESEARCH METHODS

In terms of objectives, the research is characterised as descriptive; in terms of procedures, it is survey research; and in terms of the approach to the problem, it has qualitative and quantitative characteristics. The human resources used were undergraduate nursing students at the Universidade do Oeste de Santa Catarina - UNOESC, as well as teaching staff. The theme seeks to meet the prerogatives of the Pedagogical Project of the Nursing Course, through multi/interdisciplinary practice, promoting multiple dialogues between the Structuring Teaching Nucleus, course collegiate and students, in order to provide innovative teaching practices in the health area, as well as stimulating research, logical reasoning and learning in a meaningful way on the part of the students.

This activity involved around 70 per cent of the curricular components of the Nursing course, involving all stages of the course, totalling 174 students. The Intervention Project was carried out by the 7th stage of the course. The activity was devised at a meeting with the NDE and the Nursing course collegiate body at the Unoesc Joaçaba Campus, involving the teaching plan at the start of the semester for the curricular components and culminated in many activities, such as the presentation of a Realistic Simulation - Simulated Jury, PBL (Problem-Based Learning), round table discussion, among others. The theme used was chosen by the course committee - Mental Health, which analysed a fact involving a case with national repercussions concerning the situation of nursing.

For three months, each curricular component involved sought to discuss and analyse the case across the board, reading articles, seminars, discussions, among others, as well as teaching methodologies in which the students actively participated in the process.

The presentation in the form of a mock jury, role play and round table was carried out by the seventh year students, while the other year students were responsible for analysing and judging the case.

a) Involved in the Intervention Project

There was a workshop for the teachers via the Pedagogical Advisory Service and the course coordinator, who will train the teachers in Role Play and Realistic Simulation in February during the institution's Continuing Education Week. Soon afterwards, before the start of the semester, there was a meeting of the course's collegiate body, together with the NDE of the Nursing course, where the proposal was presented to the teachers, as well as agreeing with the teachers in their Teaching Plans all the activities pertinent to the Intervention Project.

The Nursing course coordinators drew up a project for the Academic Week, where the Intervention Project activities took place.

### b) The Course's Commitment to Intervention

It is worth mentioning that it was agreed at a collegiate meeting with each teacher of each component, and that around 70 per cent of the curricular components were involved in this intervention project.

## 2.1 MATERIALISING THE PROJECT

### a) History and Rationale

The 7th stage nursing students were given the following context in which to develop a role play, round table discussion and mock jury.

> Alisson, the only child of Mrs Alzira, a single mother. The young man is 22 and autistic.

In time:

Autism is a global developmental disorder characterised by three fundamental features:

* Inability to interact socially;
* Difficulty in mastering language to communicate or deal with symbolic games;

* Restrictive and repetitive behaviour pattern.

The degree of impairment varies in intensity: it ranges from milder conditions such as Asperger's syndrome (in which speech and intelligence are not impaired) to severe forms in which the patient is unable to maintain any kind of interpersonal contact and has aggressive behaviour and mental retardation.

He was diagnosed at the age of 9. After repeating first grade three times, his mother decided to take him out of mainstream school. When the boy turned 15, with the help of the local social services, his mother agreed and offered to enrol him in a special needs school. Since then, Alisson's behaviour has worsened, becoming increasingly aggressive. At the school, there is an exclusive teacher, in an exclusive environment, with very routine and repetitive routines.

In time:

* Having a person with severe forms of autism at home can throw the whole family off balance. That's why everyone involved needs specialised care and guidance;

* It's essential to find a way or technique, no matter what it is, that makes it possible to establish some kind of communication with the autistic person;

* Autistic people find it difficult to cope with change, no matter how small, so it's important to keep their world organised and within a routine;

* Although the current trend is to include students with disabilities in mainstream schools, the limitations that the disorder causes must be respected. In some cases, it's best to look for an institution that offers more individualised care;

* High-achieving autistic people can perform like geniuses in certain areas of knowledge.

Shortly before Alisson's 18th birthday, he came home from school, became completely angry and aggressive when he saw his mother with her hair down and wearing an outfit he didn't know she was wearing. Alisson struck her three times with a knife, hitting her left arm, chest and skull. Alzira died before help arrived.

b) Intervention

The intervention took place in three stages, the first of which, after discussing the case, was for the students to do a 15-minute role-play. The second was a round table of health professionals. The third was a realistic simulation - a mock jury and a final debate on the treatment for the case.

# CHAPTER 3

# LITERATURE REVIEW

## 3.1 ANDRAGOGY AND NURSING EDUCATION

When entering the field of teaching and learning in the Nursing course, it is necessary to point out some positions that clarify how adults learn, thus revealing the importance of innovative practices in undergraduate courses, in the use of active methodologies, that is, pedagogical practices that allow the student to act on the object of knowledge.

Ferraz etal. (2004, p. 6) state that andragogy is based on four basic pillars, related to the peculiarities of adult learners, whom we take to be mature individuals, namely: (a) their self-concept develops from a position of dependence to that of a self-directed human being; (b) they accumulate a growing body of experiences that become a rich source of learning; (c) their readiness to learn makes them increasingly task-orientated with potential for development in their social role; (d) their time perspective changes from a later application of knowledge to immediate application, adapting their orientation in the sense of a change from a focus on the object to a focus on performance.

Knowles (1980) also states that it is up to the learning facilitator to check which assumptions are appropriate for a given situation. When learners are dependent, when they have no previous experience in the area, when they don't understand the relevance of certain content to their daily tasks, when they need to accumulate knowledge quickly in order to achieve certain performances; then the pedagogical model is the most appropriate.

Responsibility for higher education in Brazil lies with the Secretariat for Higher Education (SESu), which is a unit of the Ministry of Education responsible for planning, coordinating and supervising the process of formulating and implementing the National Higher Education Policy. SESu supervises private higher education institutions, in accordance with the National Education Guidelines and Bases Law (LDB) (SESu, 2014).

Based on this legal argument for higher education, it is possible to begin a process of reflection on nursing education in Brazil as the training of critical and reflective individuals, capable of acting in an integral way in society, meeting the demands of the contemporary world, which is constantly asking for competences and skills in health professionals.

The LDB, in Chapter IV, supports higher education, describing the essential characteristics for higher education professionals such as reflective thinking, insertion in professional sectors, research and scientific investigation, aiming at the development of science and technology, promotion and dissemination of knowledge to society in parallel with the provision of specialised services to the community, establishing a reciprocal relationship.

According to Zanotti (1996):

> Education will play an essential role in shaping the future of nursing, being paramount in preparing professionals as clinical nurses, administrators, educators and researchers worldwide, as well as improving the quality of nursing care.

Santos and Romanowski (2004, p.2608-9) mention that "we need to relearn how to teach by first learning how to learn", or even that

> [...] metacognition opens up new perspectives for the study of individual differences in school performance, since it emphasises the personal role in cognitive evaluation and control. Individuals with identical intellectual capacities can have different levels of academic achievement due to the way in which each one acts on their own learning processes.

Nursing is a major player in society, and this purpose gives us the idea that knowledge is a tool for building competences and skills in today's nurses. The insertion of knowledge for academics through multidisciplinary human health disciplines shows that "around and at the base of each scientific discipline, there are a number of rules, principles, mental structures, instruments, cultural norms, and/or norms that organise the world" (ROCHA; PERDIZ et al. 2007, p.23).

## 3.2 ACTIVE METHODOLOGIES

In recent decades, many changes have taken place in the educational process, i.e. the way students construct learning, where the teacher has become the mediator of knowledge.

In this sense, Vygotsky (2003, p. 298) points out that

> Until now, the student always rested on the teacher's efforts. They looked at everything with their eyes and judged with their minds. It's time for them to use their own feet and realise that the teacher can teach the pupil very little knowledge, just as it's not possible for a child to learn to walk through lessons, nor with the most careful demonstration of an artistic gait by a teacher. The child must be encouraged to walk and fall, to suffer the pain of injuries and to choose the direction. And what is true of walking - that you can only
>
> learning by doing and falling - can also be applied to all aspects of education.

It is therefore the teacher's responsibility to mediate in formal education, since students bring with them their own knowledge and the teacher's fundamental role is to enable the development of new knowledge. It is assumed that the student is an active subject and participant in the teaching and learning processes, as well as a basic element of the school environment, and that the teacher's responsibility is to contribute to the integral, full, critical, autonomous and reflective formation of each student.

In order to do this, it is necessary to analyse the organisation of the school curriculum, as it must be constructed in such a way that it corresponds to the social reality of those involved in the educational process. Sacristán (2000, p. 170) points out that "the curriculum is the expression of the social function of the school institution, and this has consequences for the behaviour of both pupils and teachers". With this in mind, managers, teachers, parents, the community and pupils must all be involved in the process. It is the school's duty to clear up any doubts and make itself understood about the changes that have taken place in educational dynamics, with the aim of improving its pedagogical practices, making the classroom an educational space in which there is interaction between teachers and students and, in this way, they build the process of acquiring knowledge, developing competences and skills.

The Law of Guidelines and Bases of National Education no. 9394/96, as well as the National Curriculum Parameters, in 1998 allowed for greater flexibility in the content to be developed in the classroom, in order to reduce the fragmentation of the disciplinary curriculum.

This new vision of reality [...] is based on the awareness of the state of interrelatedness and essential interdependence of all phenomena - physical, biological, psychological, social and cultural. This vision transcends the current disciplinary and conceptual boundaries [...]. There is currently no well-established conceptual or institutional framework to accommodate the formulation of the new paradigm, but the guidelines for such a framework are already being formulated by many individuals, communities and organisations that are developing new ways of thinking and establishing themselves according to new principles (CAPRA, 1982, p. 259).

Fazenda (2002) presents interdisciplinarity as a practice of integration, characterised by "the intensity of exchanges between specialists and the degree of real integration of disciplines within the same research project". "Three essential elements are present in interdisciplinarity: the articulation between the fields of knowledge constituted by the disciplines; the interaction between specialists; and the place where the interaction and articulation take place."

Curriculum matrices should be built on the basis of descriptors that cross curricular objectives and mental operations (competences and skills). According to (PESTANA, 1999, p.9), the matrices conceptualise competences, saying that the competences assessed are cognitive ones, which are broken down into instrumental skills. Cognitive competences are understood to be the structural modalities of intelligence, actions and operations that the subject uses to establish relationships with and between the objects, situations, phenomena and people they want to know. Instrumental skills refer specifically to "knowing how to do things" and derive directly from the structural level of competences acquired and transformed into skills (PESTANA, 1999, p.9).

Continuing teacher training is therefore essential to this process. Teachers must be in constant training, Freire (1996, p. 23) points out:

> [...] teaching is not just about transferring knowledge and content, nor is training the action by which a creative subject gives form, style or soul to an indecisive and complacent body. There is no such thing as teaching without discipline; the two explain each other and their subjects, despite the differences that characterise them, are not reduced to the condition of object, one of the other. Those who teach learn by teaching and those who learn teach by learning. Whoever teaches, teaches something to someone.[...] Teaching doesn't exist without learning and vice versa.

The notions of deformation, trajectory and teaching are intertwined when we try to understand the teacher as "the subject of their own life and of the educational process in which they are one of the actors" (ISAIA, 2003, p. 241).

Pimenta (1997), when discussing teaching knowledge, considers that teachers are formed from the needs and challenges of teaching practice. In other words, they are formed through their knowledge of experience which, when treated reflexively, underpins their hypotheses, theories and conceptions of teaching. Pérez Gomes (1995, p.104) also states that "when the professional is flexible and open to the complex scenario of interactions in practice, reflection-in-action is the best learning tool".

The pedagogical practices adopted by teachers in the process of mediating knowledge should focus on meaningful learning, based on problem-solving, problematising facts or situations in order to bring students' understanding of the fact studied.

According to Masetto (2010), active methodologies are learning situations planned by the teacher in partnership with the students that provoke and encourage participation and an active and critical attitude towards learning.

In this way, the methodologies presuppose greater and more effective interaction between students and teachers, where there is an exchange of ideas and experiences on both sides and in some cases the teacher puts himself in the student's position, learning with them.

The different philosophical, political and educational perspectives and the influences of the political, social and cultural contexts of each culture and era contribute to the existence of a diversity of approaches or "schools of thought" on assessment. However, in this work, the perspective adopted on assessment is related to operative testing and no longer just transcripts.

As Vasconcellos (2005, p.22) says, "[...] assessment plays a decisive role in reversing the situation of school failure; however, if it is based on the wrong foundations, it not only fails to fulfil its function of helping, but also becomes a hindrance to change."

Changing assessment implies changes in assessment itself (its content, its form and its intentionality), as well as in the aspects with which it is linked: pedagogical practice as a whole (pedagogical link, content and methodology of working in the classroom).

If tests have to be drawn up, they should be done well, achieving their real objective, which is to check that relevant content has been learnt in a meaningful way (MORETTO, 2005, p. 96).

Thus, healthcare-specific simulation is an attempt to reproduce the essential aspects of a clinical scenario so that when a similar scenario occurs in a real clinical context, the situation can be managed easily and successfully (JEFFRIES; MCNEILIS; WHEELER, 2008, p. 471 apud SANTOS; LEITE, p. 553). Simulation, as a safe training method, is increasingly used to train health professionals in all curricular components, but there is a lack of evidence of the effectiveness of simulation training in nursing education (ALINIER et al., 2006, p. 361 apud SANTOS; LEITE, p. 553). The learning that takes place in clinical and skills laboratories can be of high quality because students have the time and willingness to make mistakes and learn from them in a safe, simulated environment (GODSON; WILSON; GOODMAN apud SANTOS; LEITE, p. 553).

Realistic simulation is the most advanced training method in the nursing learning environment. Supported by high technology that reproduces real-life experiences through clinical scenarios, its aim is to guarantee safety in the patient care process. Using simulators, mannequins, actors, among others, in facilities that create a situation very close to the real thing, realistic simulation trains professionals in the entire patient care cycle: arrival, procedures, results, relationships with family members and the multidisciplinary team.

The connection between nursing and simulation is historical, with evidence of this relationship dating back to the beginning of the 20th century, when mannequins were developed to represent the process of caring for human beings. Despite the great initial distance between the simulated environment and the real one, this teaching format became popular and entered academic curricula globally, being widely used to this day.

According to Fonseca (2011), researchers and teachers in the health field have noticed the need to improve these teaching techniques, presenting new theories for their applicability and leading to learning from a more reliable and realistic perspective. Thus, the reconstructed and updated simulation has had its traditional concept reformulated, being recognised as a set of techniques designed to recreate, in a substitutive and comprehensive way, a working and therapeutic space that allows the learner to participate.

When they enter the learning environment, students experience the moments when nurses intervene with patients, coming into contact with them and their entire social environment in various problem situations.

## 3.3 HEALTH EDUCATION

According to EducaSaúde (2015a), discoveries in neuroscience and cognitive psychology about learning processes, the volume and transience of the knowledge base needed in health practice, access to health for people and communities, as well as greater access to health information and people's awareness, have changed expectations and requirements for health schools, forcing them to review the teaching-learning situations and environments made available to students in their academic and professional training.

In this context, for EducaSaúde (2015a), the relationship between professional training, protocols and guidelines in the area of health; teacher protagonism and participation in the pedagogical process and in the university's interactions with society, including affirmative action and social inclusion measures aimed at democratising higher education and the health system and access to education and health for minority groups.

It is through development and knowledge based on the integration of teaching and service in the management of change processes that professional training in health takes place.

Through the texts and materials available during this trajectory, the importance of the proposed objectives of this specialisation can be seen, thus strengthening the construction of a pedagogical teaching-learning process that questions the forms of power that constitute it, emphasising the socio-cultural character present in the construction of concepts and conceptions that involve being healthy-healing-healing; knowing and problematising the national historical accumulations in medical education and nursing education as social movements on the basis of the National Curricular Guidelines for Health - DCN/Saúde.

The problematisation of the lessons learned in Collective Health for changes in the education of health professionals is to interpret the correlation between the Brazilian health reform and changes in the graduation of health professions, which we have felt in very significant instances in our practice.

This will provide an interdisciplinary debate on the practices of interaction between teaching and health services in the context of changes in undergraduate teaching in the area of health; a reflective analysis of the profile of professional competences and skills indicated by the DCN/Health as "general competences and skills and specific competences and skills" and on the notion of field and core of professional knowledge and practices in the construction of multiprofessional and interdisciplinary practices of Integrality in health.

Many training institutions still adopt what is known as "hospital-centric" teaching, where specialities are the priority, while others have made an effort to move in the direction of the system, prioritising teamwork and comprehensive care. But we can't say that this happens in 100 per cent of training, although the curriculum is close to ideal, since we depend on people, spaces and many interests involved in these relationships.

When it comes to "enabling experiences" to improve learning, it's also about minimally making people aware of the health system in force, where, after all, we are inserted in one way or another. In other words, these are potentials that can be used in different spaces of interaction between the service and teaching, since the SUS organic law itself states that the system is responsible for organising the training of human resources to work in the health area (EDUCA-SAÚDE, 2014b).

Another aspect worth emphasising is the importance of using discussion spaces for training, not just those that offer services, but also those that discuss how they work, for example, we can mention the importance of putting health students in touch with councils (CMS, CLS), commissions (CIES, CIB), among others.

In short, it's clear that creating "ideal" spaces for training health professionals is by no means the best alternative, but rather putting them in constant contact with real society, real spaces where services are offered and discussions take place, in order to bring training and service closer together and ensure that they are professionals who are aware of the health system in force in the country.

Indeed, learning, teaching and training is no easy task and if we think about how many people are involved in achieving each of the items presented in the curriculum design proposal, it becomes even more challenging.

"The teacher's intentionality, articulated with their pedagogical and didactic choices, reflecting on choices in the fields of planning, curriculum, teaching strategies and learning assessment, is one of the fundamental aspects of the training proposal presented here." (EDUCA- SAÚDE, 2014b). We realise that health training is a real challenge, but I would also add the needs of the teacher, who is often "put" in the classroom without having even thought about it. Many are health (care) professionals and for one reason or another they become teachers and sometimes end up passing on the knowledge they learnt during their own training or acquired during their professional lives.

There is no ideal training proposal, what exists are ideas, actions, projects, and why not say dreams for training that takes into account intersectorality, interdisciplinarity, integration between teaching and service. I believe that proposals such as the one presented in this course for training teachers to work in health training are very significant initiatives, and will certainly take these discussions into the training institutions. (EDUCA-SAÚDE, 2014b)

Comprehensiveness indicates health care that respects diversity, people's autonomy, their beliefs, their concept of health, among other issues, and management that recognises all these issues when working/planning interventions and policies based on the territory. One of the principles of the Unified Health System, and perhaps the one with the greatest difficulty in being effective, and health care based on care networks makes it possible to get closer to it. When we read about and discuss networks, it's important to think that although they have been mentioned by the policy in its principles since law 8080/92, they have started to appear on the agenda since they were organised and defined in the policy. Certainly, the discussion of networks centred on primary care is important in the construction of the SUS and the consolidation of this policy. (EDUCA- SAÚDE, 2014b)

As mentioned in the text, it indicates that understanding comprehensiveness in health services presupposes processes in networks for its realisation. In this sense, understanding comprehensiveness in two dimensions: in the context of the health service itself, taking as a reference the care and production of care in this environment; and taking as a reference the articulation of this specific service. (EDUCA-SAÚDE, 2014b)

How can we actively use the legal precepts contained in this text and many others to present/rediscover the SUS with students, usersThe text also discusses social control, which needs to be

strengthened, the HEI, through representation on public policy management councils, is taking an important step forward, as well as encouraging students and teachers to recognise and participate in these spaces. (EDUCA-SAÚDE, 2014b)

It's worth emphasising that the discussion about training needs to take place in local spaces and with teachers who are committed to learning that combines theory and practice, and with "meaningful" experience in practical spaces where workers are also committed to training. This all leads us to think about the challenges that the course proposes and whether our proposed intervention will make these advances possible. (EDUCA-SAÚDE, 2014b)

As a strong point, it brings up the link between education and health, reviewing the history of public policies in the different sectors and how they intersect. This leads to a major reflection on how to transform these policies into pedagogical practices that will be able to train professionals with a profile for the world of work that is set out in the current health system. It also provides an important reflection on the fact that the DCN itself is still fragile in terms of professional training and the lack of depth in fields that are not specific to the health area, but which are very important when we think of participatory professionals who are capable of exercising their own citizenship, among other things. (EDUCA-SAÚDE, 2014b)

In addition, the importance of the teacher in the general context of training, after all, there is no point in an integrated curriculum, public policies that intertwine if in the daily life of the classroom, the teacher maintains repetitive pedagogical practices that are not integrated with the service and are not committed to the SUS.

There are many possible reflections based on the text and health teaching institutions need to promote this reflection in different ways. After all, teachers are one of the important players in the search for training that develops human beings in an integral way so that they can become professionals in the same way.

## 3.4 AUTISM SPECTRUM DISORDER

Autism spectrum disorder (ASD), better known as autism, is a developmental disorder characterised by alterations present from a very early age, typically before the age of three, with a multiple and variable impact on prime areas of human development such as communication, social interaction, learning and adaptability (MELO, 2007, p.17).

According to the CDC (Centre of Diseases Control and Prevention), in the USA in 2010, one in every 68 children was diagnosed with autism spectrum disorder, as shown in the following graph. (AUTISM MAGAZINE, 2014).

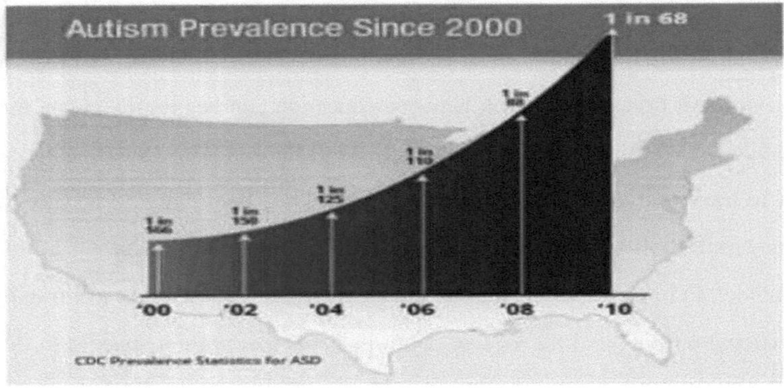


Graph 1 - Prevalence of Autism
Source: Autism Magazine (2014)

In Brazil, according to the magazine Autismo: informação gerando ação (2011), ASD affects one in every 62 children, totalling approximately 2 million people, affecting four times more males than females (MELO, 2007, p.17). According to Ferreira (2008, p. 29), girls tend to be the most affected. In the state of Santa Catarina, according to a study by Ferreira (2008), the prevalence is 1.32 autistic people for every 10,000 people, with a sex ratio of 1.23 to 1.89

boys for every girl.

### 3.4.1 Etiology

The causes of autism are unknown. It is believed that the origin of autism lies in abnormalities in some part of the brain that has not yet been conclusively defined and is probably genetic in origin. In addition, it is recognised that it can be caused by problems related to events that occurred during pregnancy or at the time of childbirth (MELO, 2007, p.17). As for genetics, "genetic studies have shown an increased risk of autism recurring: approximately 3 to 8 per cent in families with an autistic child". (GADIA; TUCHMAN; ROTTA, 2004, p.88).

Ferreira (2008) mentions that early disturbance of interpersonal relationships, due to problems of lack of affective contact with parents or other members of the child's social circle, together with a combination of organic factors such as epilepsy and convulsions, are also considered causes for a person to develop autism. Miranda (2005 apud FERREIRA 2008, p. 26) describes "maternal rubella, congenital blindness and deafness, phenylketonuria, encephalitis, meningitis and tuberous sclerosis" as predisposing factors for autism. But he adds that there is no consensus on the causes of autism. Some studies have found that autistic individuals often have compromised immune systems (CAYCEDO, 2006, apud FERREIRA 2008, p.27).

This impairment can be genetic and/or environmental, such as exposure to chemical products, which can predispose a child to autism. Another example is exposure to environmental factors such as the triple viral vaccine or vaccine preservatives containing mercury, i.e. Thimerosal (JAMES et al 2007; CHOWKA, 2002, apud FERREIRA, 2008, p. 27).

### 3.4.2 Symptoms and Manifestations of Autism

Autism can manifest itself from the first days of life, but it is common for parents to report that the child went through a period of normality before showing symptoms.
According to Cunha (2011, p.28), there are some cardinal symptoms that help recognise the disorder, which to be diagnosed requires at least eight items to be met: □ Retreat and isolation from other people

Not maintaining eye contact

□Resist physical contact

□ Resistance to learning

□ Not showing fear in real danger

□ Acting deaf

□ Tantrums

□ Not accepting a change of routine

□ Using people to pick up objects

□ Physical hyperactivity

□ Disorganised agitation

□ Too much calm

□ Attachment and inappropriate handling of objects

□ Circular movements with the body

□ Sensitivity to sounds

□ Stereotyping

□ Echolalia (repeating sounds)

□ Not being interested in make-believe games.

□ Compulsiveness

Melo (2007, p.19) also reports that 30 per cent of autistic people suffer from epilepsy. Cunha (2011, p.28) explains that this manifestation occurs because autism can be accompanied by neurological and neurochemical problems.

Gadia, Tuchman and Rotta (2004) mention some of the diseases associated with ASD, which are listed in the following table:

Table 1-Pathologies potentially associated with autism

| **Congenital/Acquired** | **Genetic/Metabolic** |
|---|---|
| Rubella | Chromosomal disorders (Fragile X, etc.) |
| Toxoplasmosis Cytomegalovirus Moebius Syndrome | Tuberous sclerosis<br>Neurofibromatosis<br>Amaurosis congenita de Leber |
| Hypomelanosis of Ito | Phenylketonuria |
| Dandy-Walker Syndrome | Histidinaemia Ceroid |
| Cornelia de Lange Syndrome | lipofuccinosis Coeliac |
| Soto's Syndrome | disease Purine metabolism |
| Goldenhar Syndrome | disorders |
| Williams Syndrome Microcephaly | Adrenoleukodystrophy<br>Duchenne muscular dystrophy |

| Hydrocephalus<br>Joubert syndrome Encephalitis/Meningitis<br>West syndrome Lead poisoning Cerebellar<br>medulloblastoma surgery | Angelman Syndrome |
|---|---|

Source: adapted from Gadia, Tchman and Rotta (2004)

### 3.4.3 Pathophysiology

According to Gadia, Tuchman and Rotta (2004, p. 87), the autistic person's central nervous system has some characteristics that differentiate it from healthy people:

□ The cells of the limbic system (hippocampus, amygdala, mammillary bodies, anterior gyrus and septal nuclei) are small, which leads to a delay in the maturation of this system.

□ Decreased number of Purkinje cells.

□ A greater number of smaller and less compact mini columns than expected.

□ Cortical abnormalities that include an increase in the volume of the left lateral ventricle or bi ventricle, the presence of cortical malformations such as polymicrogyria, schizencephaly and macrogyria.

□ Hypoplasia of lobes VI and VII of the cerebellar vemiis and hypoplasia of the cerebellar trunk

□ Anatomical abnormalities in the posterior and inferior portions of the cerebellar hemispheres, involving cell loss.

□ The fusiform facial area is markedly diminished in autistic people, who tend to activate other regions (frontal, occipital).

### 3.4.4 Diagnosis

Diagnosis is based on the criteria of the Diagnostic Statistical Manual -DSM V, which brought significant changes to the classification of ASD

The previous version of the DSM had three criteria for diagnosis, while the new DSM will have only two main areas: social communication and deficits and fixed or repetitive behaviours. Language challenges are no longer considered, as the American Psychiatric Society believes that language disorders, such as speech delay, can indicate various pathologies and are not exclusive to autism spectrum disorder.

Although the definition of autism has changed, the main characteristics of the disease remain the same. Since people with all levels of autism display many of the same characteristics, they vary in the degree to which they are affected.
which they exhibit these characteristics, the new DSM-V criteria may better reflect that autism is a spectrum of, rather than a group of, distinct syndromes.

The diagnosis of autism is basically made by assessing the clinical picture, using some of the criteria described in the Diagnostic and Statistical Manual of the American Psychiatric Association, which are described in Table 2.

**A. Pelo menos seis dos 12 critérios abaixo, sendo dois de (1) e pelo menos um de (2) e (3).**

1) Déficits qualitativos na interação social, manifestados por:
**a.** dificuldades marcadas no uso de comunicação não-verbal
**b.** falhas do desenvolvimento de relações interpessoais apropriadas no nível de desenvolvimento
**c.** falha em procurar, espontaneamente, compartir interesses ou atividades prazerosas com outros
**d.** falta de reciprocidade social ou emocional

2) Déficits qualitativos de comunicação, manifestados por:
**a.** falta ou atraso do desenvolvimento da linguagem, não compensada por outros meios (apontar, usar mímica)
**b.** déficit marcado na habilidade de iniciar ou manter conversação em indivíduos com linguagem adequada
**c.** uso estereotipado, repetitivo ou idiossincrático de linguagem
**d.** inabilidade de participar de brincadeiras de faz-de-conta ou imaginativas de forma variada e espontânea para o seu nível de desenvolvimento

3) Padrões de comportamento, atividades e interesses restritos e estereotipados:
**a.** preocupação excessiva, em termos de intensidade ou de foco, com interesses restritos e estereotipados
**b.** aderência inflexível a rotinas ou rituais
**c.** maneirismos motores repetitivos e estereotipados
**d.** preocupação persistente com partes de objetos

**B. Atrasos ou função anormal em pelo menos uma das áreas acima presente antes dos 3 anos de idade.**

Table 2-Diagnostic criteria for autistic disorder

Source: Adapted from Gadia, Tuchman and Rotta (2004)

There are no specific laboratory tests to detect autism. Usually, the doctor orders tests to investigate conditions (possible diseases) that have identifiable causes and can present a picture of childhood autism, such as Fragile X syndrome, phenylketonuria or tuberous sclerosis, as well as tests to rule out visual and hearing problems. It's important to note, however, that none of the conditions present the symptoms of childhood autism in all their occurrences. Therefore, although sometimes quite strong signs of autism appear around the age of eighteen months, the diagnosis is rarely conclusive before twenty-four months, and the most frequent average age is over thirty-one months. Early diagnosis is important in order to be able to start specialised educational intervention as soon as possible (MELLO, 2007, p.24). Even when autistic disorders are properly diagnosed, i.e. using appropriate diagnostic criteria, there is considerable variation in the symptom profile, depending on the underlying aetiology (GADIA; TUCHMAN; ROTTA, 2004, p.86). For this reason, Gadia, Tuchman and Rotta (2004, p.86) state that:

> The diagnosis of autism requires a careful clinical assessment: language and neuropsychological evaluations, as well as complementary tests (for example, chromosome studies including DNA for Fragile X and neuroimaging or neurophysiology studies, where appropriate) may be necessary in specific cases, to allow us to identify more homogeneous subgroups according to behavioural phenotype and aetiology. Only in this way will we be able to gain an understanding of the pathophysiology of these disorders and establish more specific interventions and prognoses.

### 3.4.5 Therapeutic Intervention

The treatment of autism requires multidisciplinary intervention. It consists of techniques for changing behaviour, educational programmes, work and language and communication therapies, as well as the use of pharmacotherapy (GADIA; TUCHMAN; ROTTA, 2004, p.89).

Mello (2007) mentions the most common types of intervention:

-TEACCH- Treatment and education for children with autism and related communication disorders: takes into account their strengths and greatest difficulties, making an individualised programme possible, is based on the organisation of the physical environment through routines - organised on boards, panels or agendas - and work systems, aims to develop independence.

-ABA - Applied Behaviour Analysis: aims to teach children skills they don't have, by introducing these skills in stages. Each skill is taught, in general, in an individual scheme, initially presenting it associated with an indication or instruction.

PECS - Picture Exchange Communication System: Helps the child to acquire communication skills through six steps.

The use of drugs is still in its infancy and there is disagreement between different professionals, because the causes of the disorder are still practically unknown.

Many drugs are used, especially the neuropileptics represented by haloperidol, but because of their adverse effects in chronic illnesses such as autism, they should be avoided. Antipsychotics such as rispiridone can also be used to treat irritability and aggression. Aclomipramine, a tricyclic antidepressant and non-selective serotonin reuptake blocker, is effective in treating obsessive-compulsive behaviour, but its use should be limited due to the risk of arrhythmias. Buspirone is another drug used to reduce anxiety (GADIA; TUCHMAN; ROTTA, 2004, 90).

"Selective serotonin uptake inhibitors, such as fluoxetine, fluvoxamine, paroxetine, sertraline and citalopram, have been used [...] in an attempt to reduce obsessive behaviour, rituals and stereotypes [...] and are well tolerated." (GADIA; TUCHMAN; ROTTA, 2004, p.90).

Specialised care, prior to inclusion in a mainstream school, can help the child develop self-awareness, preparing them to use role models later on. There are other forms of treatment, such as psychotherapy, speech therapy, equine therapy, music therapy and others, which are carried out on a continuous and permanent basis (MELLO, 2007, p.48).

### 3.4.6 Complementary Techniques

Mello (2007, p. 43) cites some techniques that can be applied to autistic children as an excellent complement to educational treatment: -Use of the computer as a support for learning to write in children who had already learnt to read and, due to difficulties with fine motor coordination or lack of interest, were unable to learn to write using traditional teaching methods.

-The use of a computer keyboard, in which a person with autism transmits their thoughts with the help of the facilitator, who offers them the necessary physical support, facilitates communication.

-auditory technique: the child or adult listens to music through headphones, with some sound frequencies eliminated through filters, for two half-hour periods each night for ten days. This treatment helps them adapt to intense sounds.

-Sensory integration: games that involve movement, balance and tactile sensations, using touches, massages, vibrators and equipment such as swings, seesaws, trampolines, slides, tunnels, spinning chairs, large therapeutic balls, toys, clay and others. This helps the child to understand and organise sensations. In addition to autistic children, parents should also receive support from qualified professionals, especially during the diagnosis of the disorder, and they can also receive support from people close to them or who have experience with similar situations. In addition, psychotherapy, as well as other forms of therapeutic support, can be indicated to help parents understand what is happening and what they are feeling, including

harbouring common feelings such as denial, anger, rejection, guilt, frustration and resentment (SÃO PAULO, 2011, p.5).

### 3.4.7 Services for Autistic People

According to Ferreira (2008), Santa Catarina has more than 80 institutions that cater for people with ASD, represented by the following services.

Fundação Catarinense de Educação Especial (Santa Catarina Special Education Foundation): a charitable, educational and scientific institution with legal personality under public law, not for profit, linked to the State Secretariat for Education and Innovation. It has been operating since 1968 in the municipality of São José and is the benchmark institution for autism care and diagnosis in Santa Catarina.

Associations of Parents and Friends of the Exceptional - APAE: a civil, philanthropic, educational, cultural, welfare, health, study and research, sports and other non-profit association with an indefinite duration.

Associação dos Amigos dos Autistas - AMAs (Association of Friends of Autistic People): associations recognised as non-profit charities. Their main objective is to provide support to parents, as well as guidance on autistic diagnoses and possible interventions. They aim for harmonious and healthy development in order to meet basic, educational and social needs. In some AMAs, service projects are developed which seek to provide specialised care based on educational and therapeutic proposals for autistic people, integration with mainstream education for the inclusion of autistic pupils, technical support in these schools for pupils with suspected or diagnosed autism, development, treatment, problems and potential of people with autism and to promote courses and lectures in order to inform the local community about autism and the forms of medical and educational intervention.

### 3.4.8 Prognosis

According to Gadia, Tuchman and Rotta (2004, p. 91), "the prognosis of autism is variable and probably depends on the severity of the underlying etiologies."

Studies that have followed autistic people into adulthood have concluded that the prognosis is linked to the level of ability, demonstrated in ability and language tests.

The results showed that approximately 5 to 10 per cent of the children studied became normal adults and around 25 per cent achieved considerable progress with some degree of independence. The remaining 65 to 70 per cent continue to have very significant deficits and require a high level of care (GADIA; TUCHMAN; ROTTA, 2004, p. 91).

The prognosis will also depend on when the intervention programmes are started; the earlier they are applied, the greater the difference they will make and the more significant and lasting the gains they will produce. (GADIA; TUCHMAN; ROTTA, 2004, p. 91).

### 3.4.9 National Policy for the Protection of the Rights of Persons with Disorders of the Autistic Spectrum (PNPDPTEA)

Law No. 12.764, DE 27 DEZEMBRO DE 2012 established the PNPDPTEA, which includes several items linked to the rights of people with autism spectrum disorder, including: a dignified life, physical and moral integrity, free development of personality, safety and leisure, protection against any form of abuse and exploitation, access to health actions and services, with a view to comprehensive care for their health needs, including: early diagnosis, even if not definitive, multi-professional care, adequate nutrition and nutritional therapy, medicines, information to aid diagnosis and treatment, access to education and vocational training, housing, including sheltered housing, the labour market, social security and social assistance. In addition, they will not be subjected to inhuman or degrading treatment, they will not be deprived of their liberty or family life, nor will they suffer discrimination on the grounds of their disability, and they will not be prevented from participating in private healthcare plans on the grounds of their condition as a person with a disability (BRASÍLIA, 2012).

# CHAPTER 4

# RESULTS

## 4.1 REPORT ON THE ACTIVITIES INVOLVED

### 4.1.1 Involvement of curricular components

The diagram below shows the 4 phases involved in the process, how each curricular component approached the contextualisation of the case within each cognitive axis. It is worth mentioning that this was agreed at a collegiate meeting with each teacher of each component.

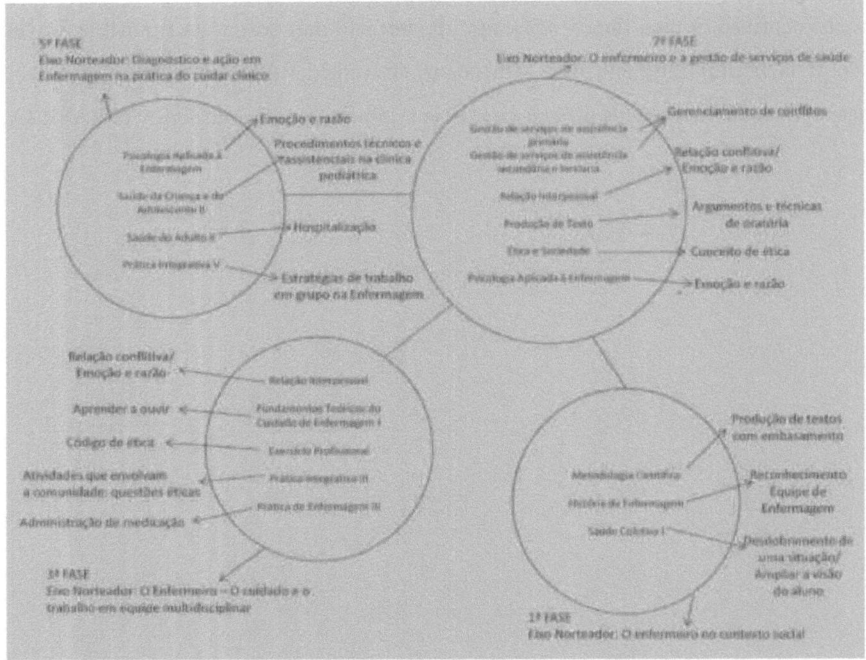


Diagram 1 - Diagram of the curricular components and their themes

It's important to note that around 70 per cent of the curricular components of the course's Pedagogical Project were involved in this activity. Diagram 1 shows the indirect involvement of the components, since only the 7th phase of the Nursing course was directly involved, especially in the Mental Health, Curricular Internship and Text Production curricular components.

Most of the curricular components addressed the context of Autism Spectrum Disorder, so that in the Round Table, Role Play and Mock Jury activities the students were aware of the subject, as well as knowing the context that would be presented and having a plausible argument.

#### 4.1.1.1 Mental Health

Historically, mental health has undergone transformations influenced by the increasingly humanitarian and holistic perceptions of both the scientific community and the community in general. In the face of such significant changes, it is essential that nurses are inserted into this context and can carry out their duties effectively. Studying the main pathologies, public policies and nursing care in mental health makes professionals prepared to act in a humanistic way in line with the new paradigm of current mental health policies in the country.

In this context, the Mental Health curricular component seeks to train nurses who are aware, humanitarian, reflective, scientifically and technologically qualified, capable of promoting, preventing and recovering mental health, facilitating the social reintegration of their clientele.

In order to develop this research project, which acted as a facilitator to achieve the objectives of the subject and the course, it was essential to interact with the other curricular components in order to combine theory and practice more effectively. Thus, the students from the 7th stage of the undergraduate nursing course took the lead in the action and, based on their structuring, the other classes acted as coadjutants, deciding in the form of a mock jury on the best course of action for the case studied.

The curricular components that centred the meetings to organise the discussion of the case were Mental Health and Text Production, where the topic of Autism Spectrum Disorder was theorised, and during the practical classes we were able to experience the practice, within the Unified Health System, of both the Nurse and the other professionals who make up the multidisciplinary team, as well as the Curricular Internship at the APAE school.

#### 4.1.1.2 Curricular Internship

According to the Federal Nursing Council, nursing is the art of caring and the science whose essence and specificity is the care of human beings, individually, in the family or in the community in an integral and holistic way, developing autonomously or as part of a team health promotion, protection, prevention, rehabilitation and recovery activities.

It is the health science that studies, prevents and treats functional kinetic disorders in the organs and systems of the human body, generated by genetic alterations, trauma and acquired diseases.

According to the Ministry of Education and Culture (MEC), the Nursing course trains professionals who are able to work in the promotion, prevention, recovery and rehabilitation of the health of individuals and the community. They work with organic dysfunctions caused by various factors, such as accidents, malformations, postural vices, neurological, cardiac and pulmonary disorders, among others. The curricular components prepare the professional to work from drawing up a physical and functional diagnosis to choosing and carrying out the physiotherapy procedures relevant to each situation, with the aim of improving the patient's quality of life by reintegrating them into activities of daily living.

The internship is fundamental to the student's training process. It allows students to showcase the learning they have acquired during the course, thus being able to integrate the subjects that make up the academic curriculum, giving them structural unity and testing their level of knowledge and understanding. Through it, students can realise the differences from the school world and exercise their adaptation. It acts as a window on the future through which we can intervene on how to apply the techniques proposed in the course syllabus in a coherent way. It should be a natural transition from knowing about to knowing, it should serve as a moment of validation of theoretical and practical learning in comparison with reality (PIMENTA; LIMA, 2009).

The internship is an opportunity for all students to experience in practice what they are learning in theory. It has the property of stimulating their critical vision for understanding and doing, and requiring their creativity and readiness to make decisions, favouring the reading of the reality of work and allowing them to identify with the activities they intend to develop as professionals.

One of the supervised internships in Nursing is Mental Health, which can be divided into two main areas: adults and children.

Some of the pathologies dealt with in Mental Health Nursing are: Patients with Paralyses, Muscular Dystrophies, Syndromes, Anoxia, Mental Disability, Hydrocephalus, Autism, among many others.

The treatment is globalised and its main objectives are: Preventing deformities, guiding the family and the patient whether adult or child, normalising postural tone, improving cognitive and memory skills, reintegrating the patient into society, reducing pathological patterns, preventing the onset of lung disease or any other complication, maintaining or increasing range of movement, reducing spasticity, stimulating activities of daily living, feeding, bladder and bowel retraining, vocational and leisure exploration; optimising the patient's quality of life (STOKES, 2000).

#### 4.1.1.3Production of Texts

Oral and written language have a definite place and importance in each individual's life, in their relationships and in influencing their competence and promotion. The pursuit of individual quality makes those interested add communication skills to their professional endeavours.

Reading texts and contexts must be constantly improved for continuous personal growth and professional information.

In this curricular component, more in-depth aspects of the text were observed, as well as the nuances of writing technical texts. It can also be observed that reading should facilitate the perception of written thought in its logic, sequence and argumentative power. Argumentation should also be observed in speech. You need to be clear about the reasons you use to make your ideas and themes clear, whether in conversation or especially in exhibitions, lectures, conferences and other contexts. Thus, public speaking, as well as knowing how to argue, are the basic principles of this curricular component.

## 4.2 SOME OF THE ACTIVITIES CARRIED OUT DURING THE PROGRAMME PHASE 7 NURSING WORKSHOPS

a) Internship at APAE School

Today, the FREI BRUNO school defines education from a perspective of broad social insertion, historically different from all the paradigms that have hitherto been used as training, technical and limited models of simple attendance. It is, therefore, a school education in which its specificities, at all times, must be geared towards the practice of citizenship. Being a dynamic school, it values and respects the diversity of the student and that they are the subject of their process of knowing, learning, recognising and producing their own culture.

It offers outpatient and semi-outpatient care to all students with a diagnosis of mental disability (moderate, severe or profound), whether or not associated with other disabilities, to children with delayed neuropsychomotor development, up to three years and eleven months, and to students with Invasive Developmental Disorders, from birth to adulthood.

The Specialised Care Service (SAESP), which is therapeutic and rehabilitative, has 11 professionals, as follows: a manager responsible for the clinic and a multidisciplinary technical team working with the students, their families and the community to provide services. The team is made up of psychologists, physiotherapists, speech therapists, social workers, occupational therapists and nursing technicians.

The internship was carried out with nursing students from the 7th phase[a] . Each group spent a week in contact with users, their families and co-workers. For the sessions we had some materials such as: medical records, cardboard, EVA, gouache paint, toothpicks, figures, guitar, costumes, music, body and oral hygiene products, body moisturiser, nail polish, sandpaper, a ball, a balloon, fruit and many others that were needed to carry out the practice.

The classroom is air-conditioned and spacious, and there is also an indoor gym and a huge outdoor patio, a well-equipped gymnasium and a tennis and ecotherapy court. All the facilities include toilets, classrooms, a library and a canteen. We catered for very dependent users who spent all day at APAE, with the use of tubes, tracheostomies and other very specific needs.

The nursing room is where all the materials needed to carry out the activities are kept, as well as a blood pressure monitor, a capillary blood glucose test and a thermometer.

In order to improve the students' performance, the institution offers workshops in various disciplines, such as handicrafts, carpentry, dance, among others, each with its own separate room and well-structured with the necessary material for their practice. The aim is to improve their performance and social interaction, as well as improving their motor coordination, emotional skills and other aspects.

The internship at the APAE Frei Bruno school took place from 18 May to 26 July 2015, under the supervision of Professor Marcia Restelatto and the assistance of Professor Eduardo Janir de Souza. The internship group is made up of students from the 7th[a] phase of the Nursing course at UNOESC. The internships ran from 7am to 11am in the morning and in the afternoon from 1pm to 5pm, following a timetable that was planned on the first day of the internship together with the students and the institution's pedagogical coordinator.

We got to know the unit, studied the medical records, gave educational talks, held study groups, worked on self-care, healthy eating, oral and body hygiene, theatre, dance, music, and provided care such as nursing consultations, specific procedures, case studies and large group discussions, as shown in the photographs below.

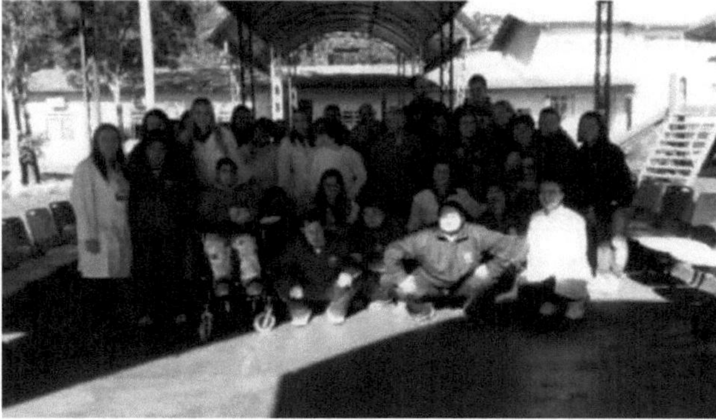

Photograph 1 - Staff, nursing students and pupils from APAE Frei Bruno

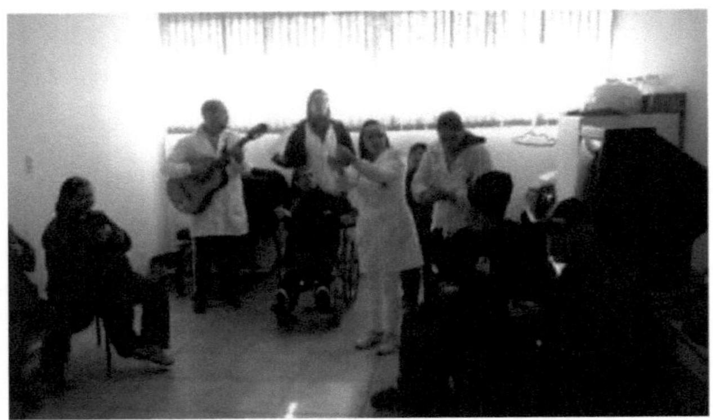

Photograph 2-Nursing students carrying out a music activity

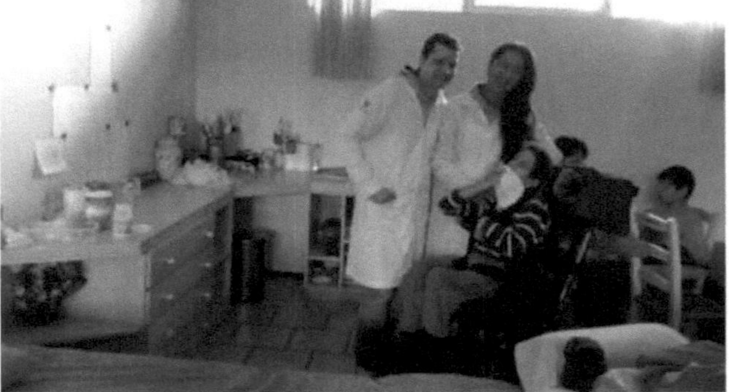

Photo 3-Nursing students carrying out a hygiene activity

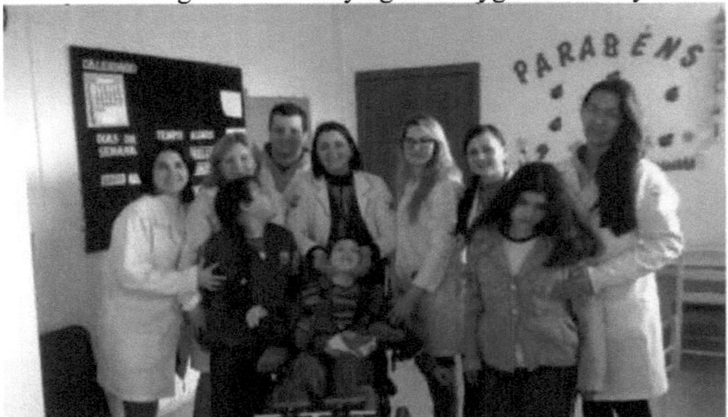


Photo 4-Nursing students and anamnesis

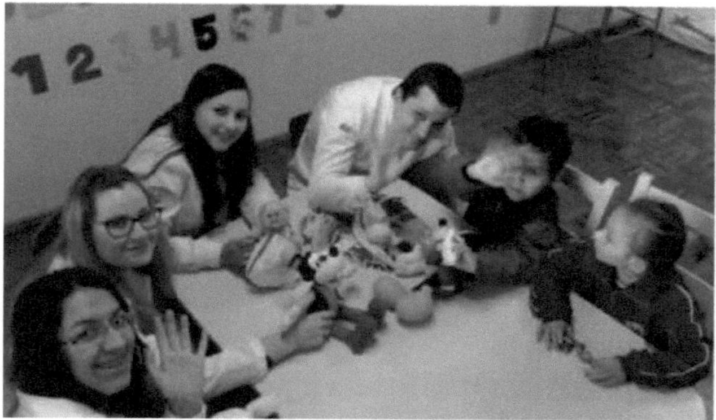

Photo 5-Nursing students developing play activities

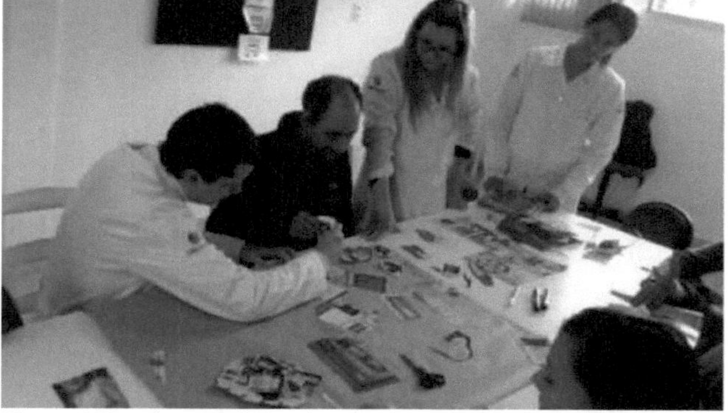
Photo 6-Nursing students developing cognitive activities

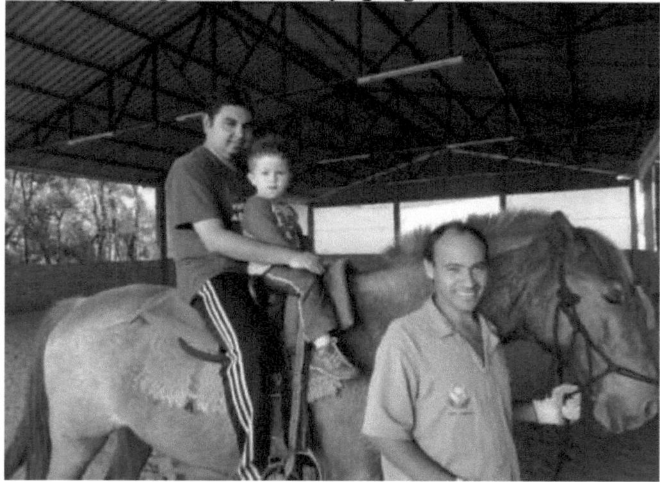
Photo 7-Ecotherapy

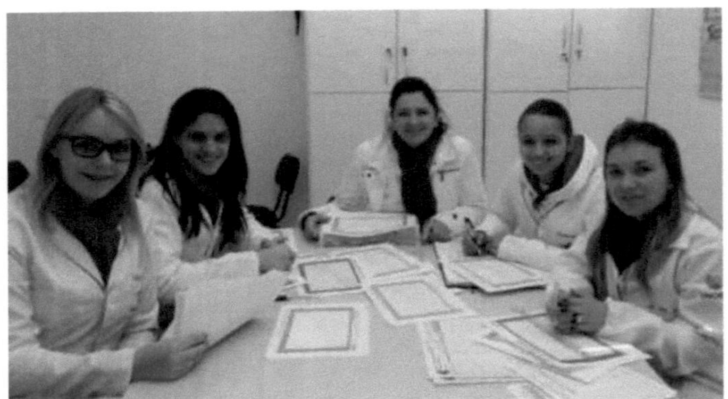

Photo 8-Nursing students analysing medical records

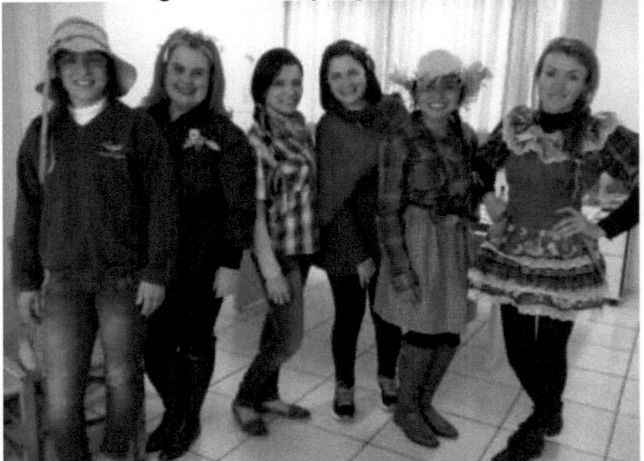

Photo 9-Nursing students and recreational activities

The Supervised Internship in Mental Health - APAE was of great importance for academic education, as the students gained experience in this area that they had not had before.

Identify that nursing plays an important role in the rehabilitation of these users, using intervention methods globally and individually according to the needs of each user, always aiming to make the patient as comfortable as possible.

It's a beautiful and exciting area to work in, where every day of my internship I've become more involved with the users due to the affection that many of them show, and the appointments end up being very rewarding.

New learnings permeated the working days, because the context of Special Education is in full change, requiring new perspectives and the search for knowledge. This is what has driven us and will always drive us, because we know that we are walking together with Education and Health to build new success stories together.

The work of habilitation and rehabilitation for people with disabilities has sometimes been misunderstood by the main policies for the care of people with disabilities, because they have a reduced view of this universe and consider that if the person with autism is being cared for in one area there is no demand in another. This fragmented way of analysing the care provided by habilitation and rehabilitation organisations and the needs of people with autism needs to be overcome, because the great thing about these organisations is the interdisciplinary approach and the multi-professional team.

People with intellectual and multiple disabilities often need care in the areas of health, education and social assistance, where each policy has its own specific action that largely benefits the disabled person. Understanding the diversity of this work has been a challenge in some spaces.

We understand that the responsibility for making public policy lies with the state and that social organisations have been partners in offering services, since the state's actions have not been sufficient to meet demand. From this perspective, dialogue between public authorities and third sector entities is of fundamental importance in the quest to improve the quality and scope of the services provided, without bureaucratic restrictions, since one of the objectives of the
APAE is social protection for vulnerable groups and is carried out in an integrated manner with sectoral policies.

b) Activities in the Mental Health Component

The need to train nurses who are suitably qualified to work in the different areas of their training, knowing how to work as part of a team, resolving conflicts and expanding their knowledge, has been evident not only because of the wide field of activity of this professional, but also because of the coordination of the health services for which nurses are generally responsible. Coupled with such responsibility, we find students interested in learning, but tired of the traditional methodologies usually employed in their training. With the aim of offering, integrating and fostering knowledge, the subject of mental health combined with the subject of text production has given undergraduate nursing students a new experience in their studies, where they have left the comfort of listening to and following classes using previously prepared material, to seek knowledge according to their real needs and interests, making learning more dependent on the student themselves.

In order to organise this activity after it had been approved by the course's collegiate body, the subject's teaching plan provided for certain moments to discuss the case.

In the second meeting of the component, the students (20 students) were divided into three randomly chosen groups. At this meeting, each group was given explanatory material about the activity to be carried out, as well as an explanatory lesson on the PBL (Problem-Based Learning) method. After the explanation, the students were asked to choose a coordinator and a secretary for each team, so that they could be the link between the groups and with the teacher.

PBL is a teaching and learning methodology based on the principle of using problems as a starting point for acquiring and integrating new knowledge, i.e. the problem comes before the theory.

Through this type of activity it is possible to develop:

* The ability to study a problem as a team;
* The ability to discuss and debate, going beyond the simple juxtaposition of ideas;
* Deepening the discussion of a topic by reaching conclusions;
* Increasing knowledge through the diversity of interpretations on the same subject;
* Have the opportunity to develop their participation in groups, their verbalisation, their team relationships and their ability to observe and criticise group performance;
* Trust that you can also learn from your peers (as well as your teacher) and value the feedback they can give you for your learning.

At first, the students' concern about the method was clear; most of them expressed feelings of insecurity and fear about how they would be assessed. The main concern when faced with the problem case was: "Professor, what do you want us to study?"

As a result, six scientific articles on the subject of autism were presented, which served as support for the emergence of key ideas and the exploration of the unknown. Each team was asked to submit a written work containing theoretical research on the knowledge acquired, and to make a video dramatising the case in role play mode.

To carry out the dramatisation, all the students were involved and built their characters based on the problem case, supported by theory and the knowledge they deemed necessary to express in the best possible way the characteristics of the person with autism spectrum disorder and all the health professionals necessarily involved in providing adequate care for this patient.

In order to bring academics closer to the reality of autism and the role of health professionals within the Unified Health System, a technical visit was organised to the Association of Friends of Autism (AMA), in the municipality of Campos Novos-SC.

AMA is a non-profit organisation that emerged in Brazil in 1983 from the interest of parents with autism in sharing information, researching the subject and improving the quality of life of their children. As a result of their efforts and those who became interested in the subject, AMA has a suitable structure for the development of specific activities for autistic people.

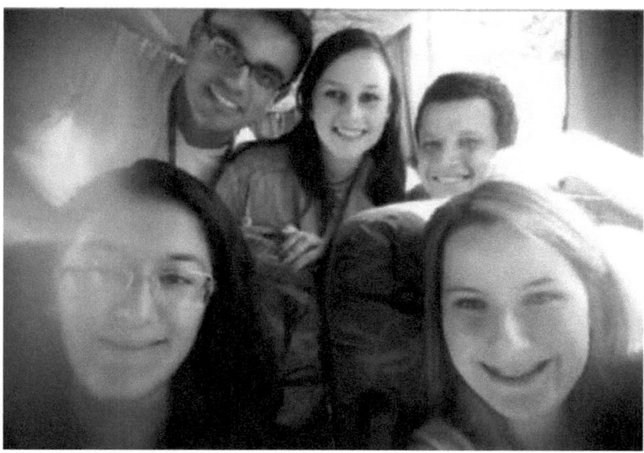

Photo 10-Technical visit toAMA

During the technical visit, it was possible for the students to have direct contact with autism and its different characteristics, as well as to share their perceptions and experience on the subject with different professionals involved in the process of caring for autistic people.

## 4.3 INTERVENTION PROJECT ACTIVITIES

a) Role Play

*Roleplay* is a teaching technique in which participants are involved in a problem situation, taking on different roles from those they experience in their daily lives, and must make decisions and predict their consequences (NESTEL; TIERNEY, 2007). According to Ruiz-Moreno (2004), this exercise is a democratic and participatory teaching methodology that addresses content and learning by understanding learning in action.

The first activity of the intervention project was a Role Play (reconstructing the facts) with the 7th stage of the Nursing course in the Mental Health curricular component. It was filmed and watched by everyone before the round table at the X ACADEMIC WEEK OF THE NURSING COURSE.

The activity had a script:

Part 1: Childhood - Characteristics of the Pathology

Part 2- Adolescence - School (APAE) , Pathology in Treatment and Interview with teacher, involvement of the Nursing service and its commitment to identifying cases. It seeks to show the context of the ESF (Family Health Strategy), as well as the commitment of the nursing professional.

Part 3- Adult - decompensated autism - murder of the mother

The result of this activity can be accessed at the following link: http://www.youtube.com/watch?v=gGNvPOmQ9Zo.

b) Round table at the X Nursing Academic Week

The second activity was a round table at the X ACADEMIC WEEK OF NURSING, on 12 May 2015.

It is worth mentioning that this was the pre-event of the Realistic Simulation - Mock Jury.

In order to make it possible to build and unite all the new concepts and perceptions about autism and to construct the role play, each class was given 30 minutes for the students to organise the activity. The role play was filmed for later presentation during the course's academic week, and from this video a round table discussion was built. The round table included academics, teachers of the mental health, supervised internship and text production components, the director of the AMA and a pedagogue and specialist in autism spectrum disorder, and listeners included academics from all phases of the nursing course, psychology academics, nursing and psychology teachers and the general public.

At this event, it was possible to present the knowledge acquired by the students, integrating teaching and health through discussion with professionals and users of the Unified Health System. The activity was widely publicised on social networks and news sites, contributing to a greater understanding by the population of autism, the SUS, and the inclusion of different health professionals, especially nurses, in public health policies. As can be seen in Photograph 11.

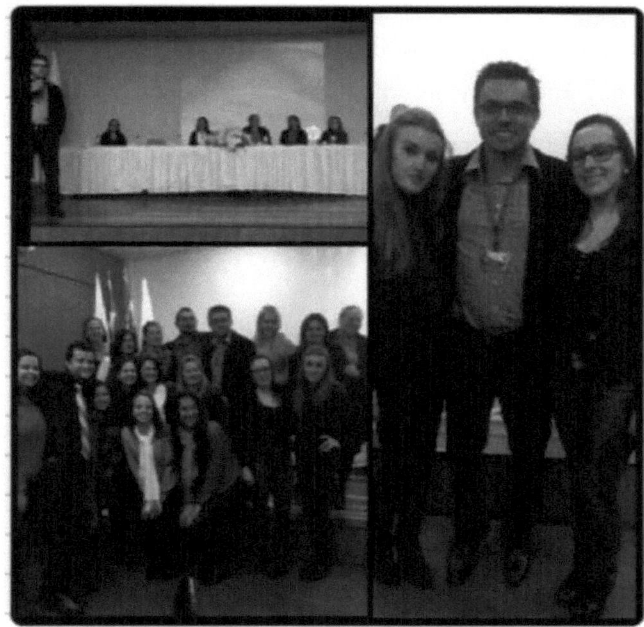

Photo 11 - Round table

The students were initially anxious about what was new, especially when they were presented with the teaching plan for role play, the problem-based research format and the mock jury.

During the course of the activities, it was possible to observe a continuous and growing interest on the part of the students in discovering and expanding their knowledge, which culminated in the success of the activity and in the professional development that was later assessed during the practical classes where these students developed activities directly with autistic people and were able to strengthen and integrate teaching-service-learning.

After this event, the students continued the activity in the Text Production curricular component, with the structuring of the mock jury. The various activities carried out in the mental health component fostered knowledge about the main topic - autism - as well as the current needs of the SUS, users and health professionals in order to improve the services provided in the public health network.

c) Realistic Simulation - Mock Jury

The third activity developed was the Realistic Simulation, presented on 26 June 2015, which the Text Production curriculum component was responsible for organising. The activity was organised on three fronts: 1-One argues that Alisson should stay with his family.

2-Another argues that he should be tried.

3- You should be referred to a care home.

The students in the other phases vote on Alisson's fate (1st, 3rd, 5th and 9th phases), as can be seen in Photos 12 and 13.

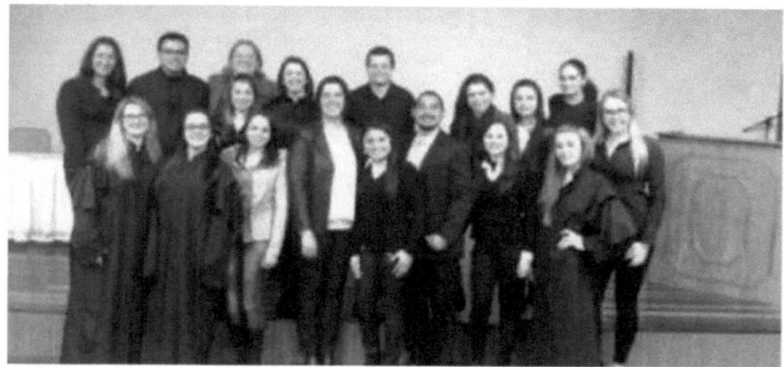

Photo 12 - Mock Jury

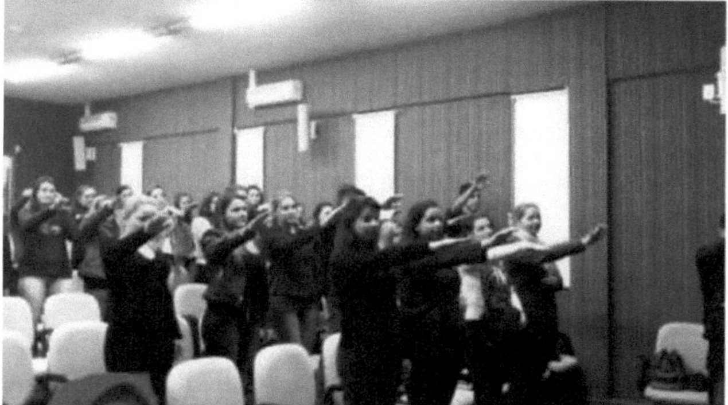

Photo 13 - Mock Jury

The activity aimed to promote a debate among those present on how to deal with the situation presented involving an autistic person. The case, based on real events, dealt with the story of a boy who, at the age of 9, began to show characteristics of autism, which were noticed at school by his teachers. His mother doesn't accept the situation and only seeks help when the teenager turns 15. At 18, something unexpected happens in the family. The mother receives a family inheritance and, with the money, decides to change her appearance. One day, when she gets home from school, her son finds the new look strange and stabs his mother to death.

As a result, it was decided at the time how to proceed with the situation. The youngster could be brought to justice for the act, sent to the care of another family member or taken into a home.

After the judgement, those present decided by vote that the autistic boy should be sent to a home where he can be given the best possible care.

# CHAPTER 5

## FINAL CONSIDERATIONS

After drawing up the project and studying the various themes in the different strands of the course, the use of active methodologies seemed to be a pleasant and effective way of working on interdisciplinarity, promoting not only health education but also professional self-knowledge.

The PBL, role-playing and mock jury activities integrated not only the nursing students, but also the community through local news reports and the students' own contact with SUS users and professionals.

According to the text Management and participatory protagonism in teaching and health work (2014), the teacher's intentionality, articulated with their pedagogical and didactic choices, reflecting on choices in the fields of planning, curriculum, teaching strategies and learning assessment, is one of the fundamental aspects of the training proposal presented here.

When I applied and proposed the activities to the students, I was extremely pleased with the results. It was possible to form new teams in the classroom, to conflict ideas, to get the shyest student interested in showing how much he knew and how much he was committed to acquiring knowledge. It was possible to get everyone out of their comfort zone and prove to them that anything is possible and that change depends more on yourself than on others.

The text Teacher protagonism in the face of training commitments to the HUS (2014) states that society recognises as professionals those individuals who solve the problems of their area using, among the technical alternatives available, those that best apply to each situation, and so the better prepared the professional is to act, the better their professional fulfilment will be. It's up to us as teachers to transform these students into outstanding professionals, and the more their critical thinking and holistic vision are developed, the greater their opportunities will be.

It wasn't easy to contain my emotion when I saw academics developing not only theoretical knowledge about autism, but also knowledge of the world and the need to value human beings.

The development of this project has provided not only knowledge about teaching in the health sector, but also different ways of teaching and learning, making students realise that the needs of human beings go beyond a pathology, that the entire social, cultural and economic context must be taken into account, that all professions are fundamental to establishing a better health condition for the patients under their care, because interdisciplinarity is essential.

I believe that the use of active methodologies, applied in this study, demonstrates good applicability, with enriching results for the academic environment, given the participation and engagement of all those involved in the process. It would still be necessary to evaluate the knowledge obtained by these academics in the long term, to understand if the knowledge was really properly acquired and if it translates positively into the practice of the professional inserted in the single health system.

The subject of Mental Health certainly gave the students a different perspective, because at first, when I presented the teaching plan and asked what they thought of the proposal, many said that it was "killing class", that they didn't have time, that it was difficult. As the classes went by, they realised that they were learning more and more, and the more they learned, the more they wanted to learn.

As a teacher of the subject, it was frustrating to hear that the proposal was to "kill a class", but the proposal was continued and the work gained notoriety and seriousness, especially on the part of the students who began to show more and more interest in doing an excellent job.

Conducting classes in the traditional lecture format is certainly more comfortable for the teacher than using active methodologies, as it requires less time to prepare and apply the content, but with the use of active methodologies it is possible to see the student active in their teaching-learning process, as it is not enough to memorise the slides, it is necessary to absorb the knowledge.

# CHAPTER 6

## REFERENCES

ADLER, S; BECKERS, D; BUCK, M. PNF Proprioceptive Neuromuscular Facilitation: An illustrated guide. 2ª Ed. São Paulo: Manole, 2007.

BRASILIA. DilmaRousseff. Presidency of the Republic - Civil House - Sub-Cabinet for Legal Affairs. LAW NO. 12.764, OF 27 DECEMBER 2012. 2012.
Available at: <http://www.planalto.gov.br/ccivil_03/_ato2011-2014/2012/lei/l12764.htm>.
Accessed on: 14 March 2015.

CASTRO, C; JUNQUEIRA, M. Pensando a terapia ocupacional em um caso de Síndrome. Cadernos de Terapia Ocupacional da ÚFS Car, 2003, vol. 11 n"I. Accessed on: 06 September 2015.
Available at:
http://webcache.googleusercontentcom/search?q=cache:PpAoXM5sHdoJ:www.cademosdeterapiaocupacional.ufscar.br/index.php/cadernos/article/download/205/160+&cd=8&hl=en-BR&ct=clnk&gl=br.

CUNHA, Eugenio. Autismoe Inclusão: psicopedagogia e práticas educativas na escola e na família. 3. ed. Rio de Janeiro: Wak, 2011. 135 pdf>. Accessed on: 14 March 2015.

FERRAZ,Serafim Firmo de Souza; LIMA, Tereza Cristina Batista de;SILVA, Suely Mendonça de Oliveira e. Learning contracts: andragogical principles and learning management tool. In: ENCONTRO DA ASSOCIAÇÃO NACIONAL DE PÓS-GRADUAÇÃO EM ADMINISTRAÇÃO-ENANPAD, 28, 2004, Salvador. Proceedings..., Salvador: ANPAD, 2004. 1 CD-ROM.

FERREIRA,Evelise Cristina Vieira. Prevalence of autism in Santa Catarina: an epidemiological view contributing to social inclusion. 2008. 95 f. Dissertation (Master's Degree) - Postgraduate Programme in Public Health, Federal University of Santa Catarina, Florianópolis, 2008. Available at: <https://repositorio.ufsc.br/handle/123456789/92166>. Accessed on: 26 April 2015.
Fonseca AS et al. Creation and implementation of the Realistic Simulation Centre of the Nursing Professional Improvement Centre: an experience report. Nursing Journal, v. 154, p. 156-160, 2011

FREIRE, P. Pedagogia da autonomia: saberes necessárias à prática educativa. 37th ed. São Paulo: Paz e Terra, 2009. 148p.

GADIA,Carlos A.; TUCHMAN, Roberto; ROTTA, Newra T.. Autism and invasive developmental disorders. Journal of Paediatrics: Brazilian Society of Paediatrics. Riode Janeiro, Dec. 2004. p. 83-94. Available at: http://www.scielo.br/pdf/jped/v80n2s0/v80n2Sa10.pdf>. Accessed on: 15 March 2015.

ISAIA, S. M. de A. Professor in higher education: weaves in the making. In: MOROSINI, M. C. (et al.). Encyclopaedia of university pedagogy. Porto Alegre: FAPERGS/RIES, 2003.

KNOWLES, M. The modern practice of adult education: from pedagogy to Andragogy. EnglewoodCliffs: Cambridge, 1980.

MELLO, Ana Maria S. Ros de. Autism: A practical guide. 5. ed. São Paulo: Ama, 2007.

MINISTÉRIO DA EDUCAÇÃO E CULTURA - MEC, Undergraduate course in physiotherapy -

proposal for curricular guidelines. Brazil, 2013. Accessed on 30 October 2013. Available at: http://portal.mec.gov.br/cne/arquivos/pdf/Fisio.pdf

NESTEL, D.; TIERNEY, T. Role-play for medical students learning about communication: guidelines for maximising benefits. BMC Med. Educ., v. 7, n. 3, p. 1-9, Mar. 2007. doi: 10.1186/1472-6920-7-3. Available at: <PMC1828731/pdf/1472-6920-7-3.pdf> PEREZ GOMES,A. The practical thinking of the teacher: the formation of the teacher as a reflective professional. In:NÓVOA, A. (Org.).Osprofessoresesua formação.
Lisbon: Publicações Dom Quixote, 1995, p. 77-91.

PIMENTA, S.G; LIMA, M. Estágio e Docência: questões e propostas. 4ª São Paulo: Cortez, 2009.

Revista Autismo: Informação gerando ação, 2011, title: Brazil stands out on World Autism Day (2 April) 2011. Available at: http://www.revistaautismo.com.br/diamundial201. Accessed on 14 March 2015.

RUIZ-MORENO, L. Group work: innovative experiences in the field of education and health. In: BATISTA, N.A.; BATISTA, S.H. (Orgs.). Teaching in health: themes and experiences. São Paulo: Senac, 2004. p.85-99.

SANTOS, L. dos and ROMANOWSKI, J. P. 2004. Metacognition: the significance of learning strategies in pedagogy courses. In: ENCONTRO NACIONAL DE DIDÁTICA E PRÁTICA DE ENSINO, 12, Curitiba, 2004. Proceedings, Curitiba, PUCPR, 12:2607-2612.

SANTOS, M. C.; LEITE, M. C. L. The evaluation of learning in the practice of nursing simulation as teaching feedback. Rev Gaúcha Enferm., Porto Alegre (RS); v. 31, n.3, p.552-6, Sep., 2010.

SÃO PAULO. Renata Flores Tibyriçá. Public Defender's Office of the State of São Paulo (Ed.). Rights of people with autism. São Paulo, 2011. 21 p. Available at: http://www.autismo.org.br/site/images/Downloads/direitospessoasautismo leitura.p

STOKES, M. Neurology for Nursing. 1st Edition, Editorial Premier, 2000.
XHARDEZ Y. KINESIOTHERAPY VADE-MÉCUM. 4th Ed. São Paulo: Andrei Editora LTDA, 2001.

FEDERAL UNIVERSITY OF RIO GRANDE DO SUL. Centre for Education, Evaluation and Pedagogical Production in Health (EducaSaúde). Specialisation Course in Teaching in Health: Management and participatory protagonism in teaching and health work. Porto Alegre: UFRGS/EducaSaúde, 2014. Support material for the Specialisation Course in Teaching in Health. Available at: https://moodle.ufrgs.br. Accessed on 10 April 2015.

FEDERAL UNIVERSITY OF RIO GRANDE DO SUL. Centre for Education, Evaluation and Pedagogical Production in Health (EducaSaúde). Specialisation Course in Teaching in Health: Teacher protagonism in the face of training commitments to the SUS. Porto

Alegre: UFRGS/EducaSaúde, 2014. Support material for the Specialisation Course in Teaching in Health. Available at: https://moodle.ufrgs.br. Accessed on 18 April 2015.

ZANOTTI, Renzo. Expanding the Frontiers of Nursing Education
Globally. Vol. 4.Ribeirão Preto - SP: Revista Latino Americana em Enfermagem.1996.

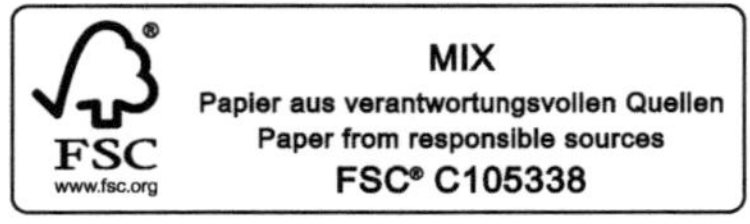


Printed by Books on Demand GmbH, Norderstedt / Germany